Stillness.

Habits to maintain mental wellness
and give *Resilience* a break

Maurya Walker Glaude, Ph.D., M.S.W., L.C.S.W.-BACS

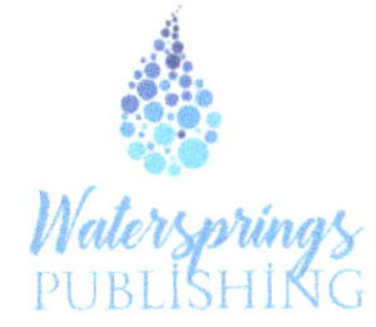

Stillness.

Habits to maintain mental wellness
and give *Resilience* a break

Stillness by Maurya W. Glaude published by
Watersprings Publishing, a division of Watersprings Media
House, LLC., P.O. Box 1284 Olive Branch, MS 38654

www.waterspringspublishing.com

Contact the publisher for bulk orders and permission requests.

Printed in the United States of America.

ISBN-13: 978-1-964972-01-5

Table of Contents

Dedication

I am grateful to my Mom and Aunt for modeling rest and resistance. Mom, I appreciate how you napped on Sundays to allow your body to rest. You not only listened to your mind and body; you showed obedience to God. And, Aunt Shelby, your frequent retreats to your boudoir demonstrated resistance to overextending your body as a hostess, wife, mother, and aunt. You modeled a balance of mental and spiritual well-being (and amazing skincare).

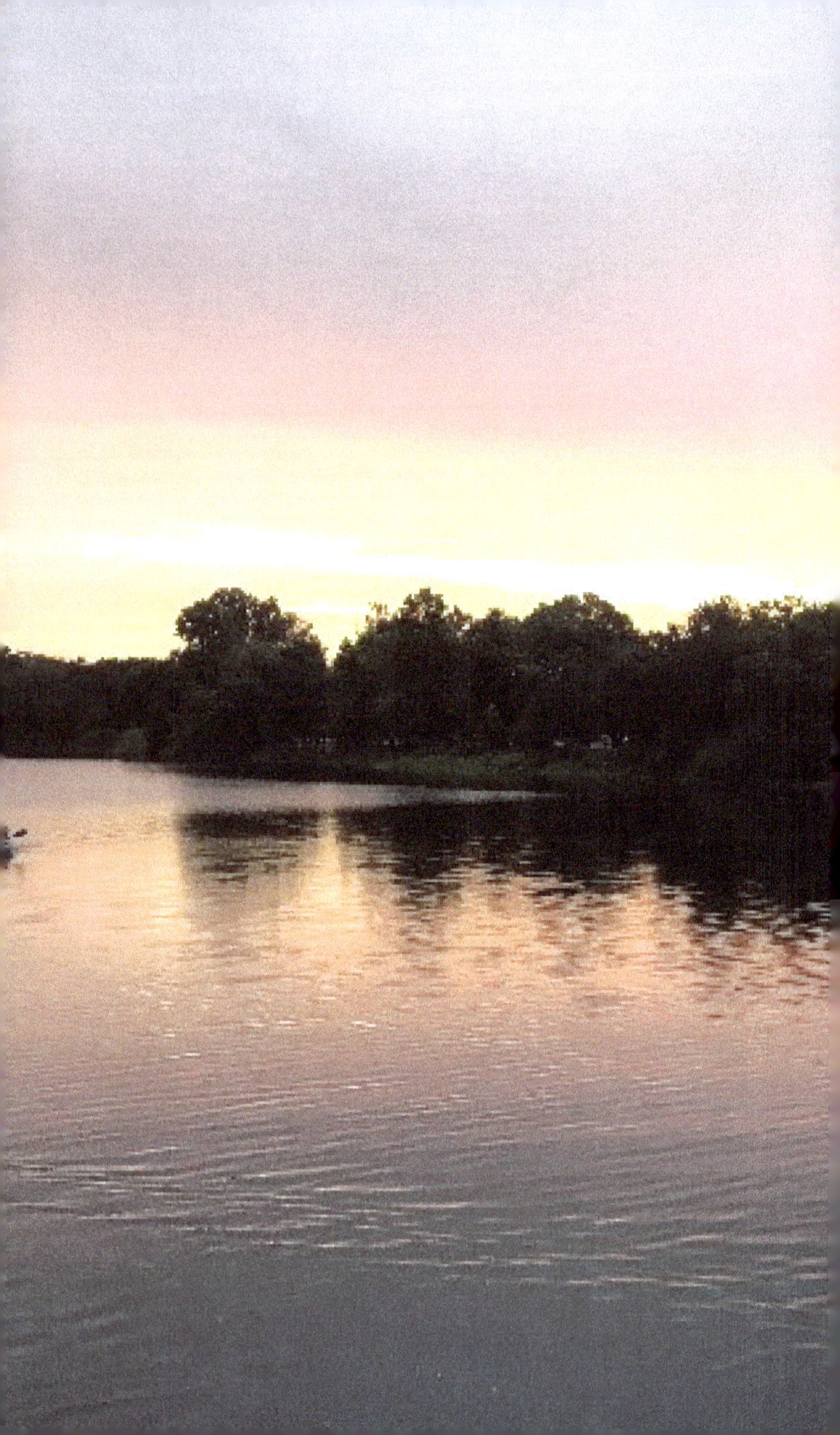

Introduction

When was the last time you were still? When was the last time you felt extreme relaxation? Whereas, you may have visited *Resilience* lately, do you remember the last time you slowed your body down enough to visit the stillness of *Serenity*? We are a generation of doers with many of us feeling overextended and overcommitted, stressed, and exhausted from constantly doing. As a society, we are socialized to think about productivity based on output, and we visualize success based on how busy we are throughout our days filled with tasks. Many of us use mental or written checklists to assist us as we navigate life's multiple identities as leaders, caregivers, parents, students, friends, volunteers, partners, and spouses. In these times, we often struggle to find equilibrium and balance in our day. We may identify feelings of fatigue, exhaustion, and hypervigilance, forcing our bodies to access mental, emotional, and physical reserves.

Our bodies naturally attempt to manage excess stressors, challenges, and demands by resourcing our sister *Resilience*. We visit her more often than we might plan to do so, and we may neglect to visit other kind souls like *Stillness, Relaxation*, let alone *Serenity*.

This book shares many seeds of wellness. This book also offers tips to help you intentionally be still to give our older sister Resilience a break. I hope you will learn or relearn some sustainable habits that cultivate wellness. Maintenance is key, and maintaining a regimen that embraces stillness will be key to longevity, wellness, and a higher quality of living.

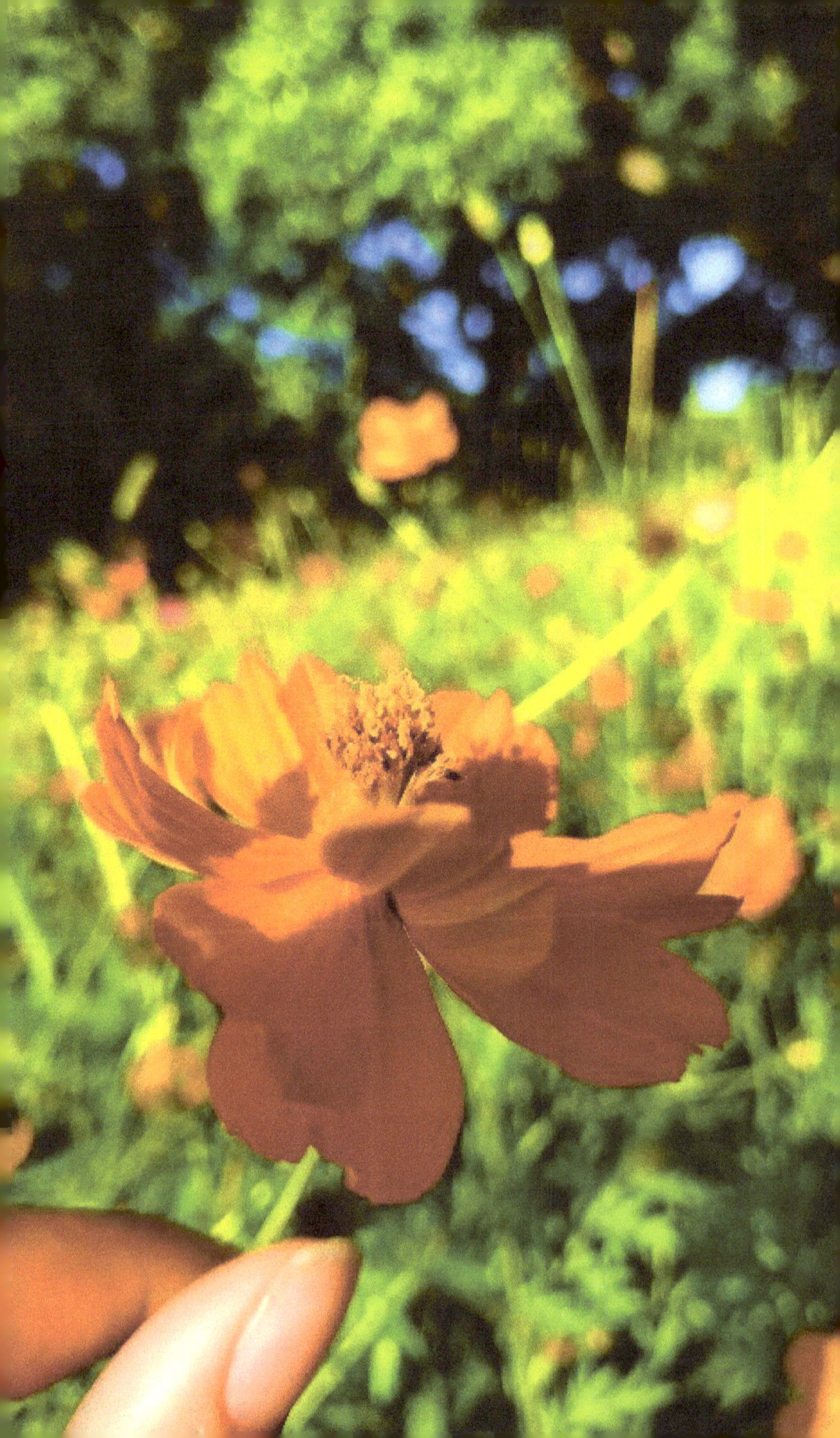

Stillness

Let's begin with *Stillness*. To be still and do it well requires us to make a conscious decision to pause.

Stillness requires us to actively participate in pausing.

For many, slowing down to be still takes too much time and planning. Being still can also demonstrate resistance. Sometimes I hear resistance from the women with whom I work in therapy. Some even try to rush through a session and not actually pause to do the work of caring for their mental wellness. Some experience shame around taking some time to care for themselves. In these moments, I demonstrate resistance through stillness. In these moments I actively listen, model patience, and invite stillness into the space while I silently ask my Higher Power to make me a vessel of hope and inspiration. Stillness is a daily decision. Will you pause and join me to reconnect with *Stillness?*

Protect some time and pause all distractions for at least three minutes.

Sit.

Stand.

Lay.

Gaze.

Notice Stillness.

Visualize Stillness.

Imitate Stillness.

What does she look like? How does she smell? How does she sound?

She appreciates when you pause to notice her.

She feels complimented when you try to look like her.

She appreciates when you intentionally stop to breathe in her sweetness.

She smiles when your energy and vibrations are in one accord.

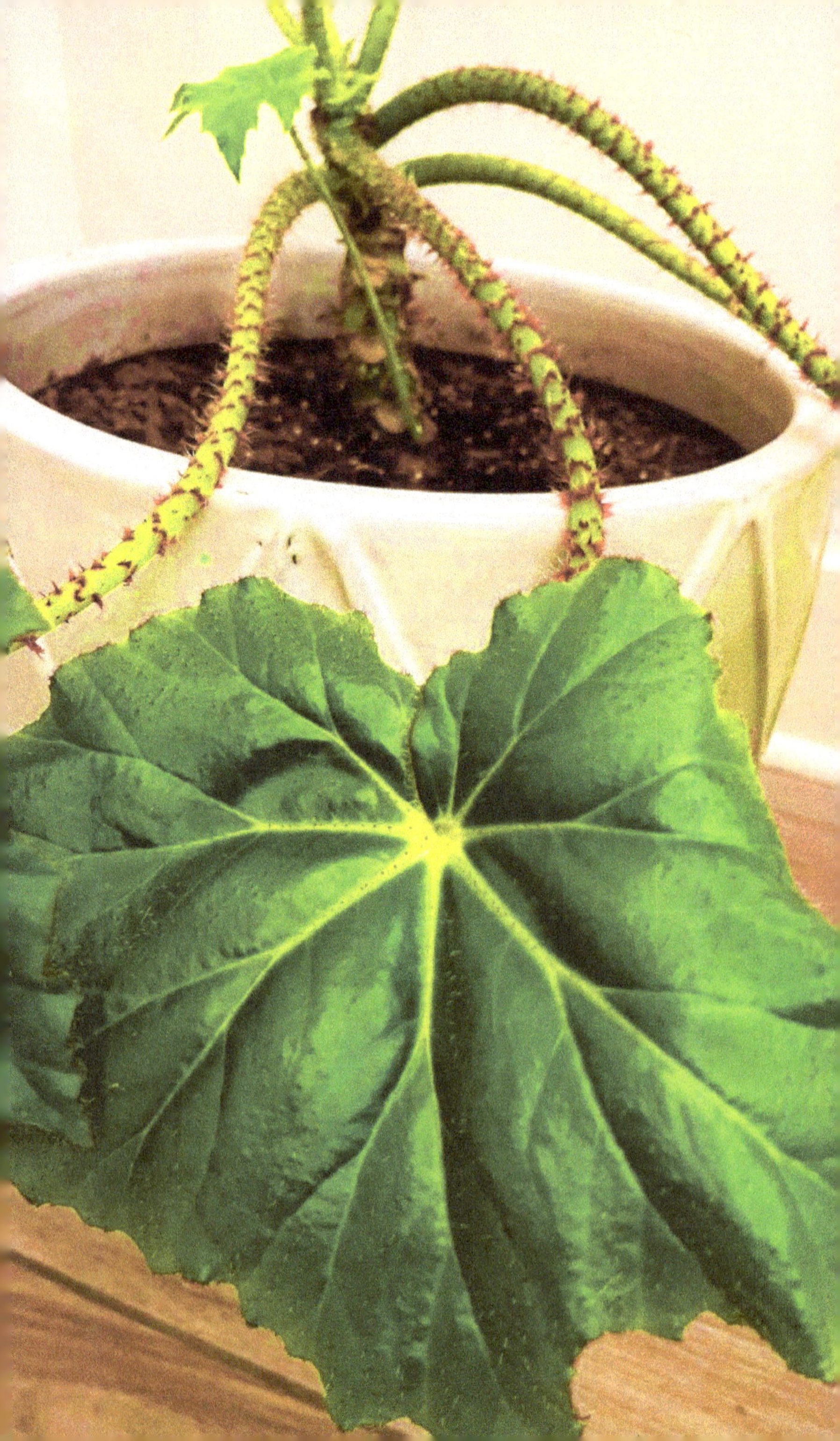

Breathing

My plant, lovingly named *Ms. Begonia*, seems to love it when I breathe. She especially seems to love it when I exhale out loud. She joined the family during the recent global COVID-19 pandemic and is a gift from a colleague who moved up north to become the Dean of a school. I learned a lot about waiting from her, I will share more about that journey later. I remember the day I replanted *Ms. Begonia* in her new pot and how nervous I was about the possibility of her adjusting poorly to her new space. She drooped and lost some stems and leaves. *Ms. Begonia* also visited her sister *Resilience* for many weeks. She also communicated her needs as we resourced energy in a reciprocal relationship. She let me know when she needed water. She let me know when she needed more light. Today, while thriving, she continues to communicate her needs very effectively. I notice how she effortlessly stretches and reaches for the light near the window where she resides. She has me very well trained and she has found a sense of balance. Similarly, our bodies communicate needs. Needs for light, touch, connection, hydration, and breathing.

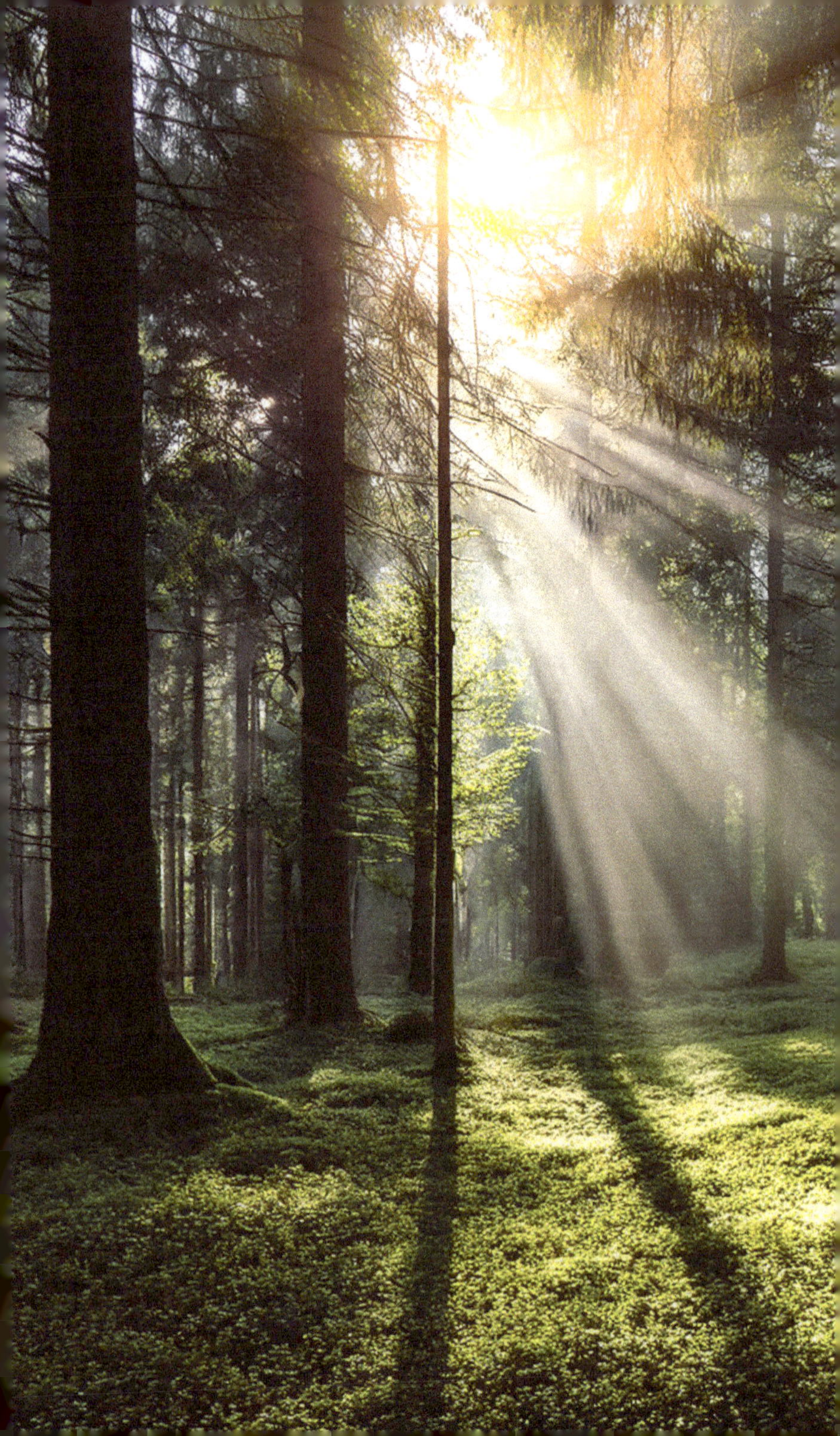

Breathing Exercise

First, focus on an image. Control your breathing and increase intentional positive thoughts.

Breathe in safety through your nose.

Exhale fear through your mouth.

Again, breathe in safety while saying, "May I feel safe. I am safe."

Exhale unsafe thoughts.

Finally, try to inhale and hold your breath for a count of three. Hold the gift of air for a count of three. Exhale while counting to three. Repeat.

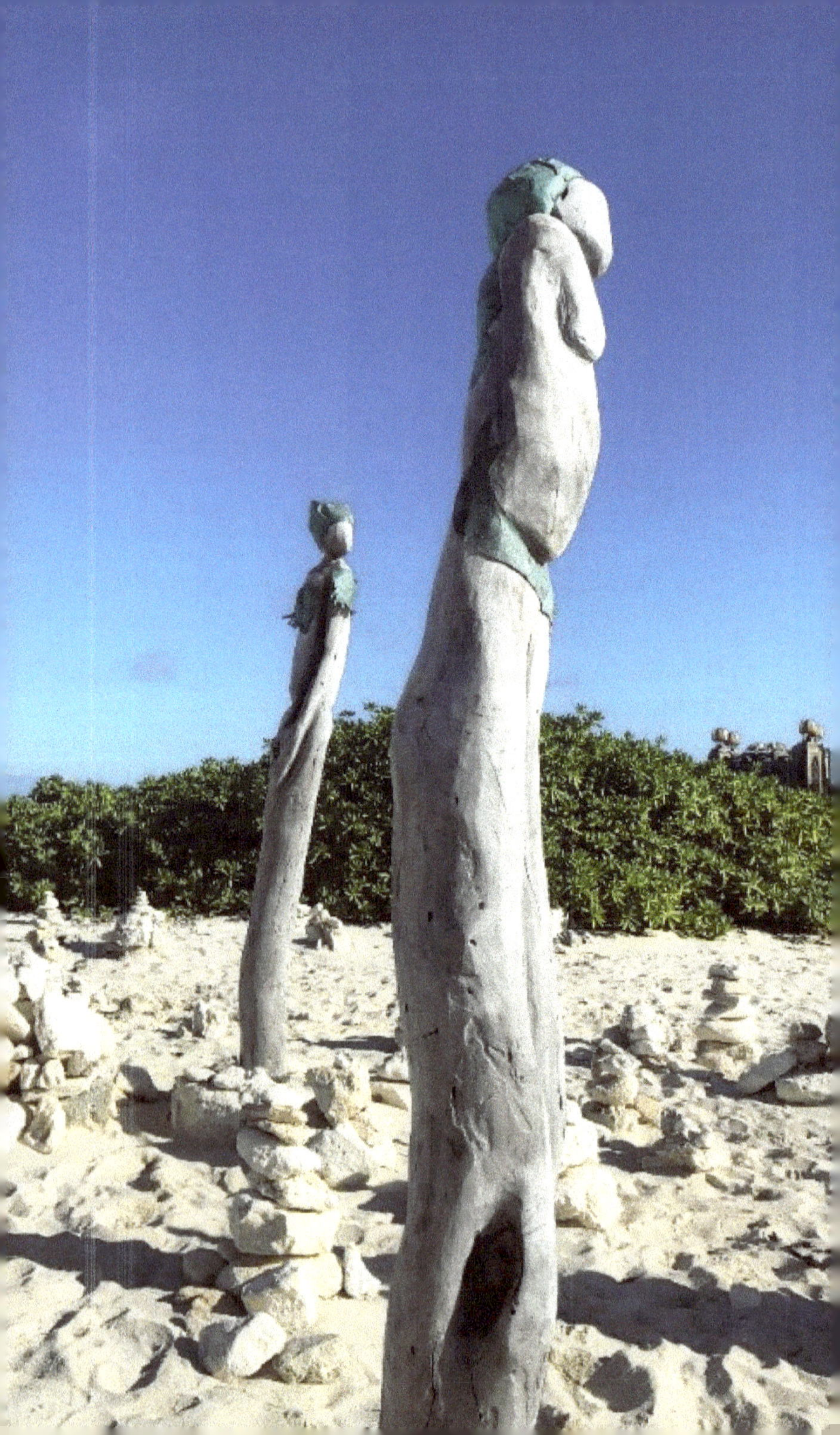

Protecting Time

Practice breathing and increasing intentional thoughts.

Breathe in safety.

Exhale fear.

Exhale unsafe thoughts.

Again, breathe in safety while saying "May I feel safe. I am safe."

Repeat.

Try to inhale and hold your breath for a count of three. Hold the fresh air for a count of three. Exhale while counting to three. Repeat.

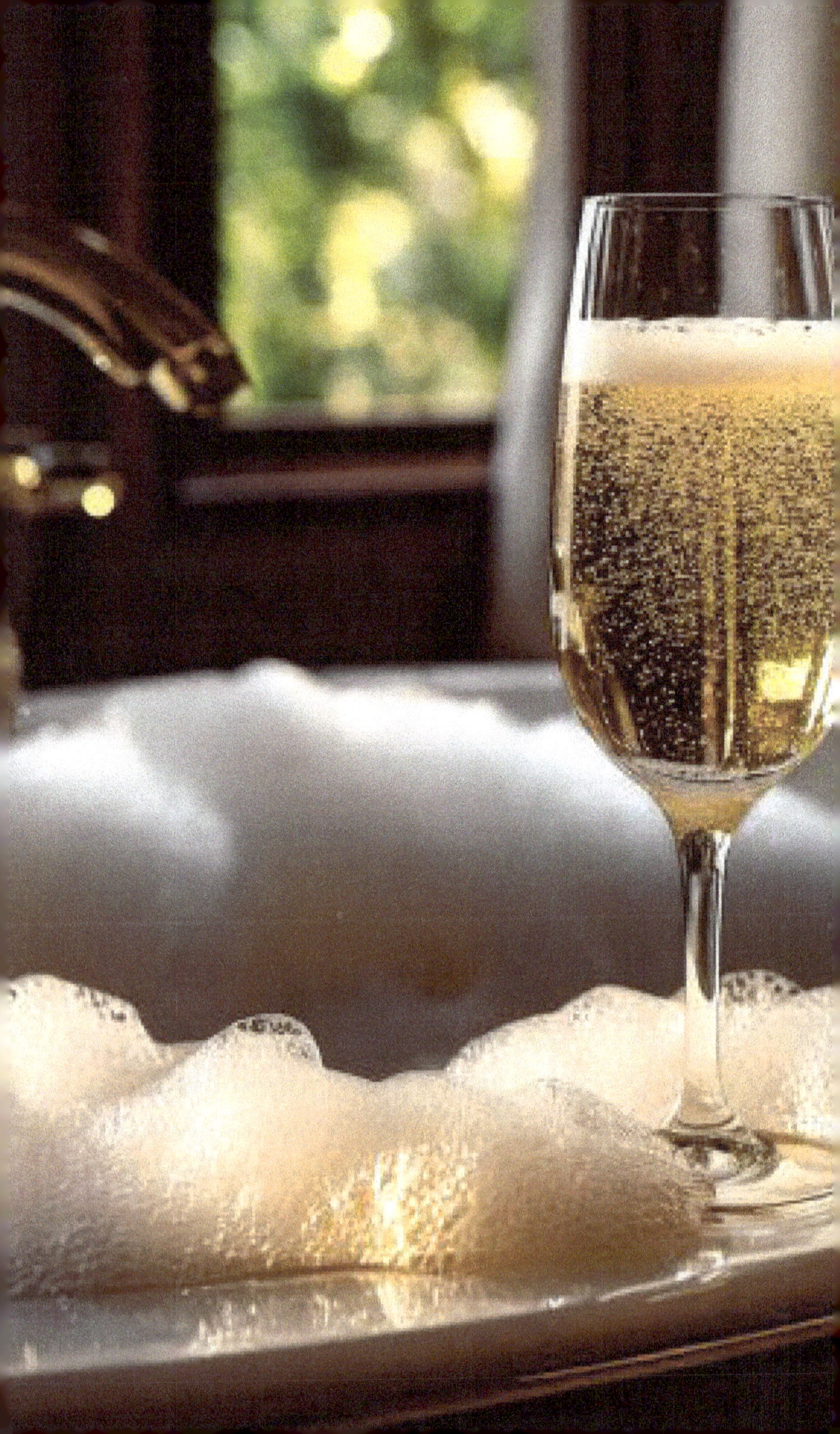

Add bubbles, like
bubble bath,
champagne,
sparkling water,
or blowing bubbles,
and practice
deep breathing.

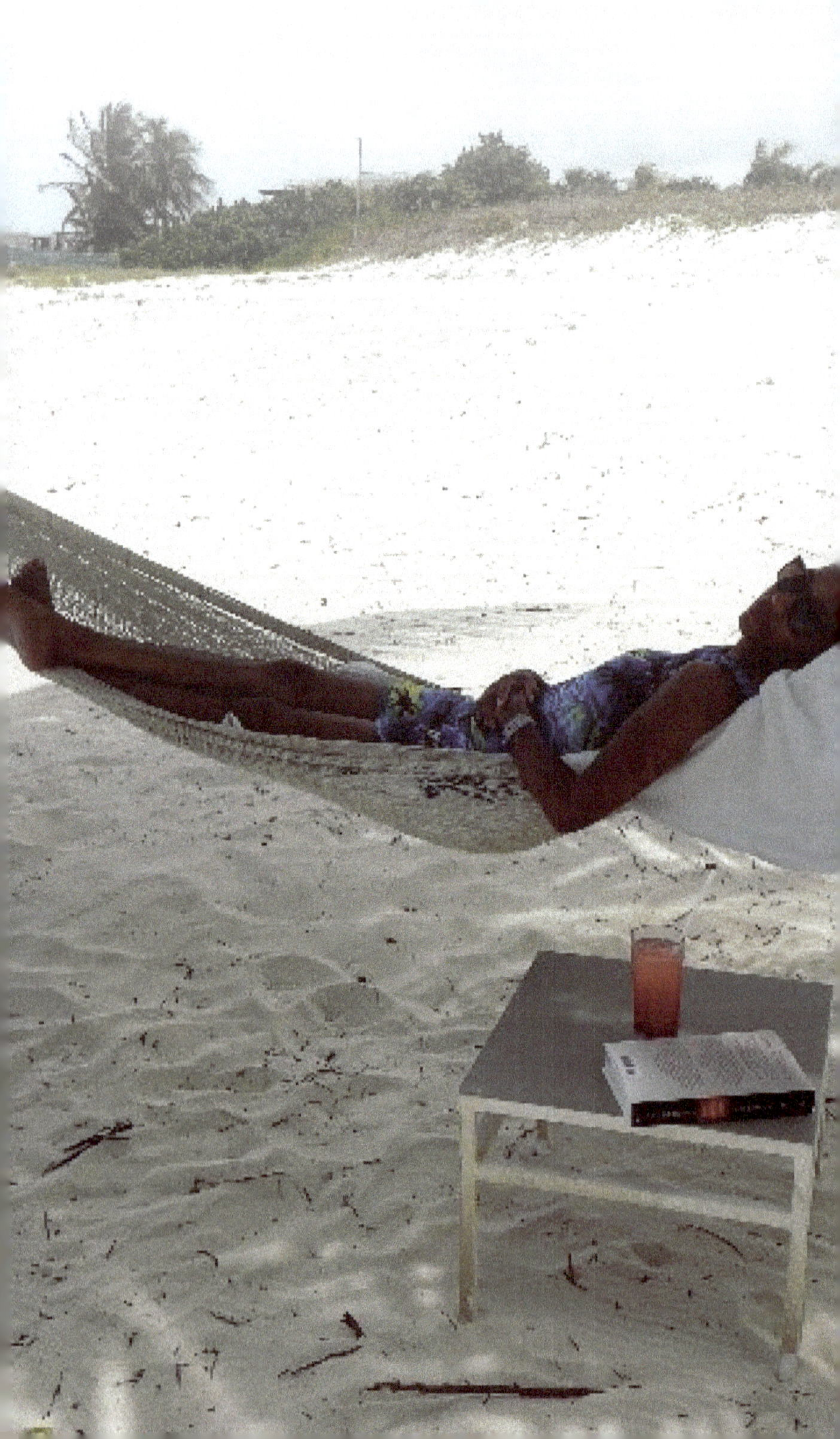

Napping

Napping is resting. Napping is resourcing. Napping is resistance. Napping gives my older sister Resilience time to rest. Rested and strong, I rise after napping. I rise, bringing the gifts and the talents that my ancestors gave me. I am their hope that rises after napping, refreshed, and filled with resources.

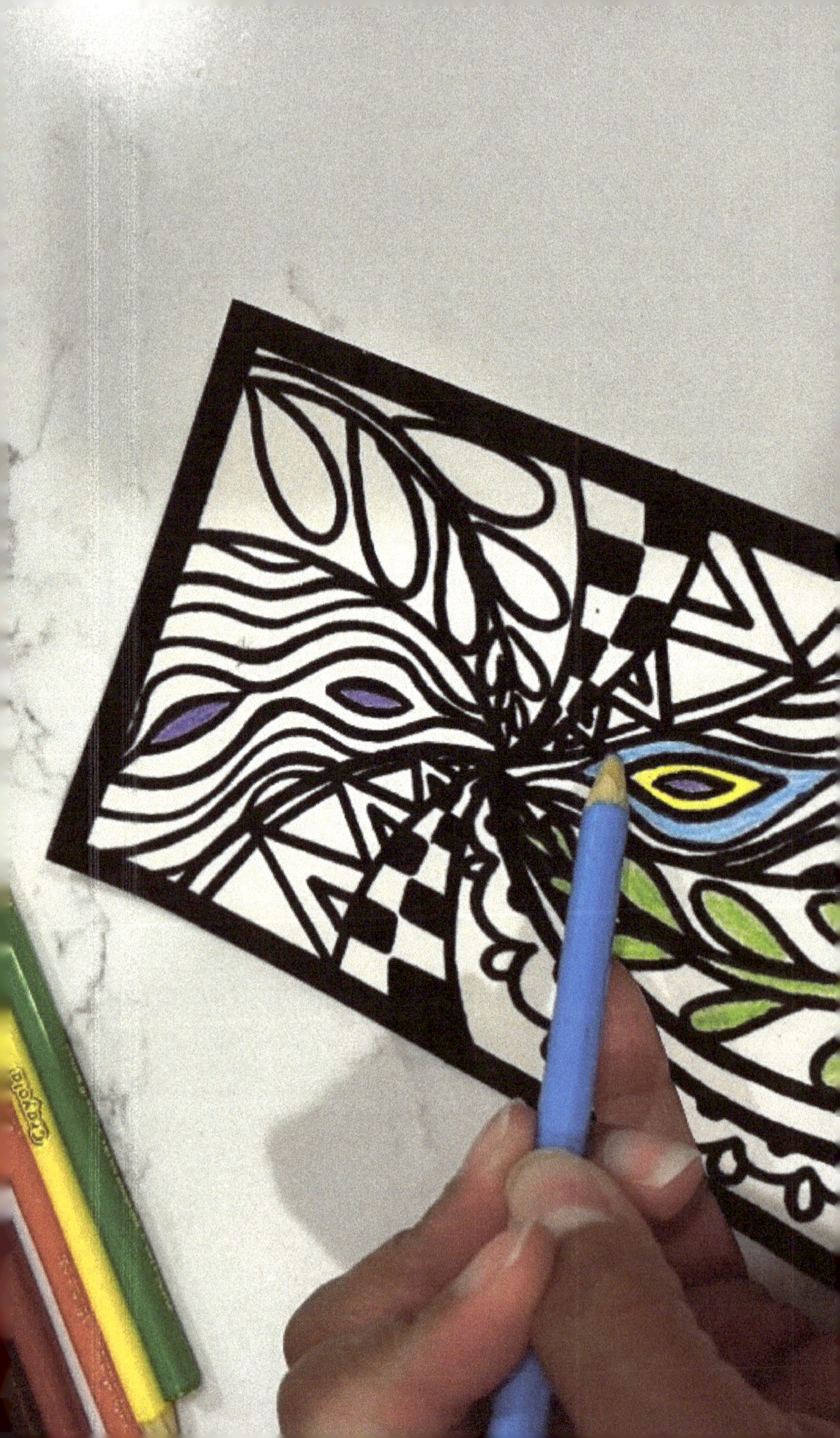

Coloring

Does the rhythm feel musical?

Does your body remember the art? Does your hand recall the pace and flow that is creating a sense of peace within?

Does your inner self remember the comforting hum and rainbow of colors?

The promise has always remained within you, and patiently your soul has awaited your return to the healing energy of coloring.

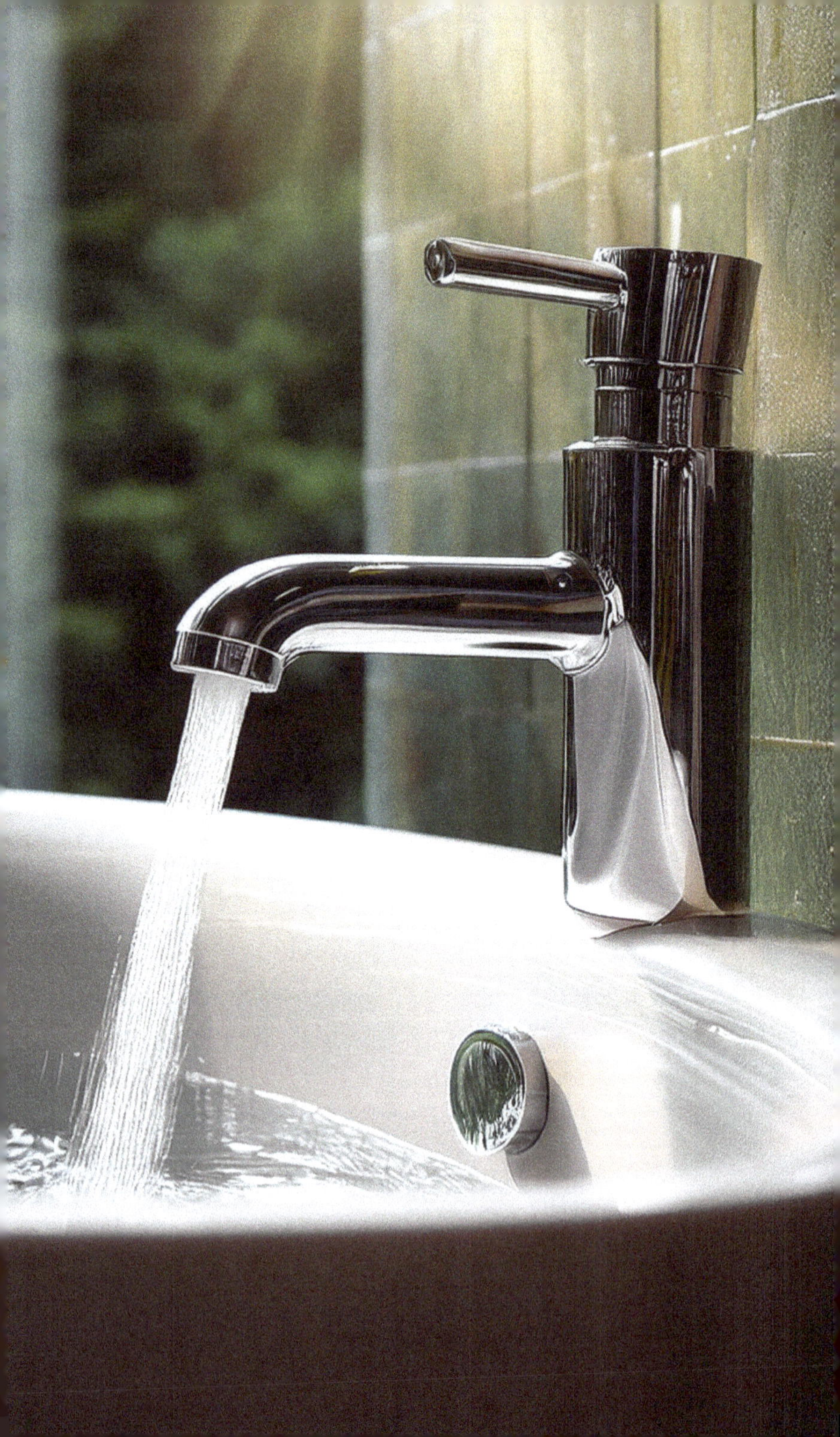

Bathing

Bathing cleanses.

Bathing cools.

Bathing warms.

Bathing is familiar.

We are reminded of the womb.

We are reminded of cleansing.

We are reminded of the refreshment of hydration.

We are reminded of our creation.

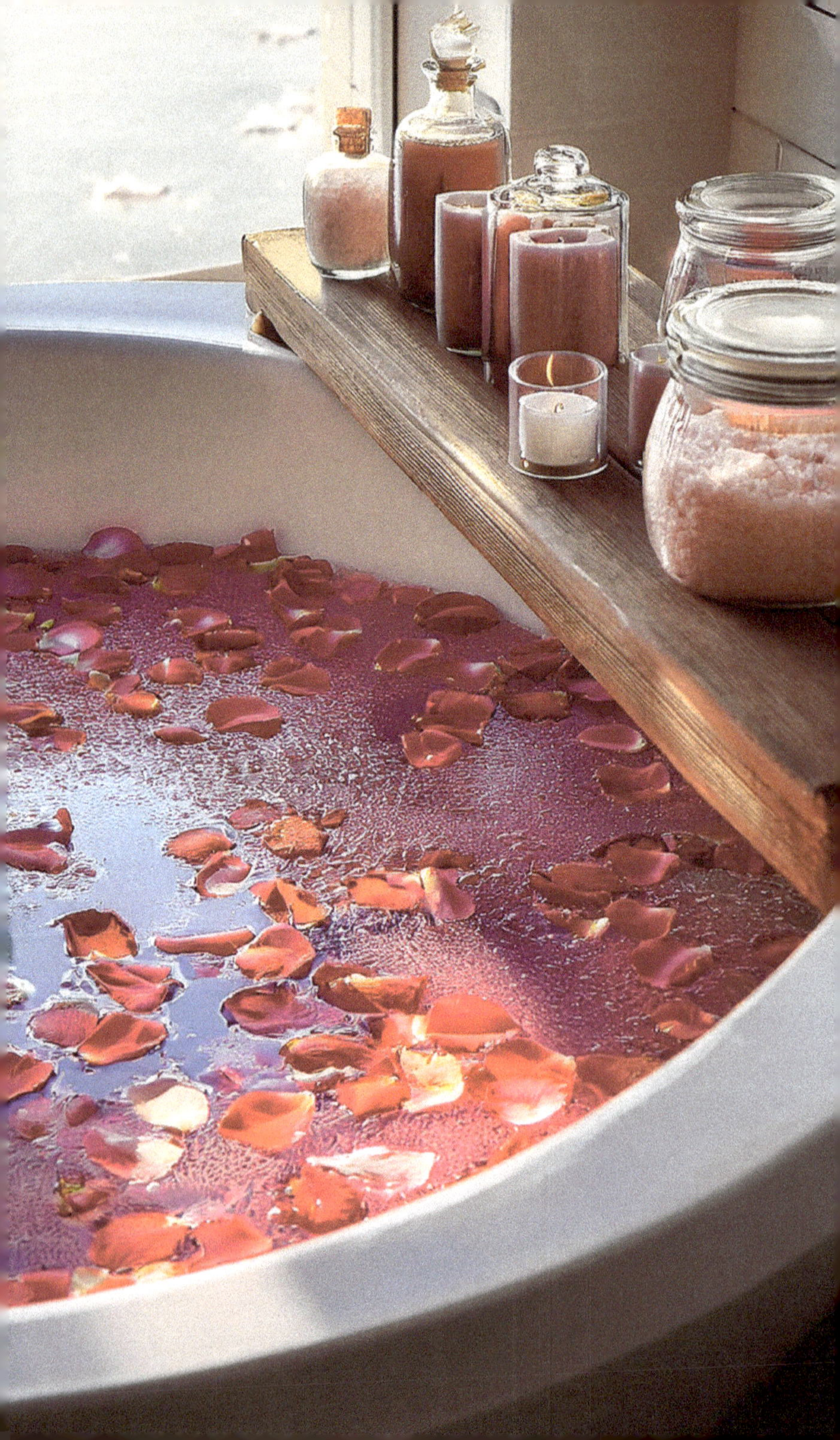

Add something
pleasurable, like
bath salts or
flower petals.

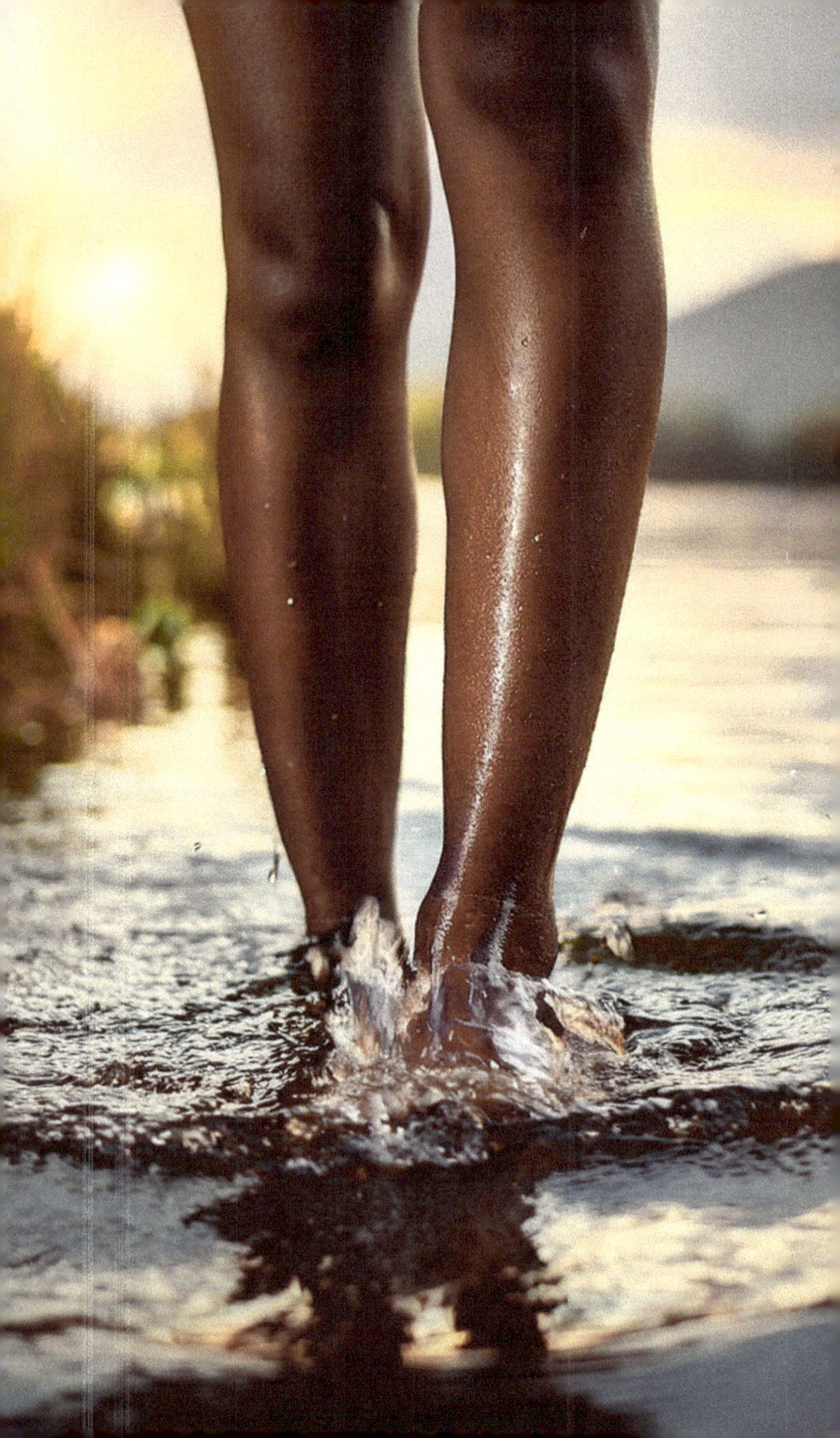

Wading

Wading began long ago. I know this because my body remembers. And, as my ancestor's chosen one, I recognize my responsibility to pause and resume wading.

Today, I wade in the ocean filled with the tears of my mothers.

Today, I wade to cleanse my body of the sweat from my labor.

I wade to comfort my body and refresh my soul.

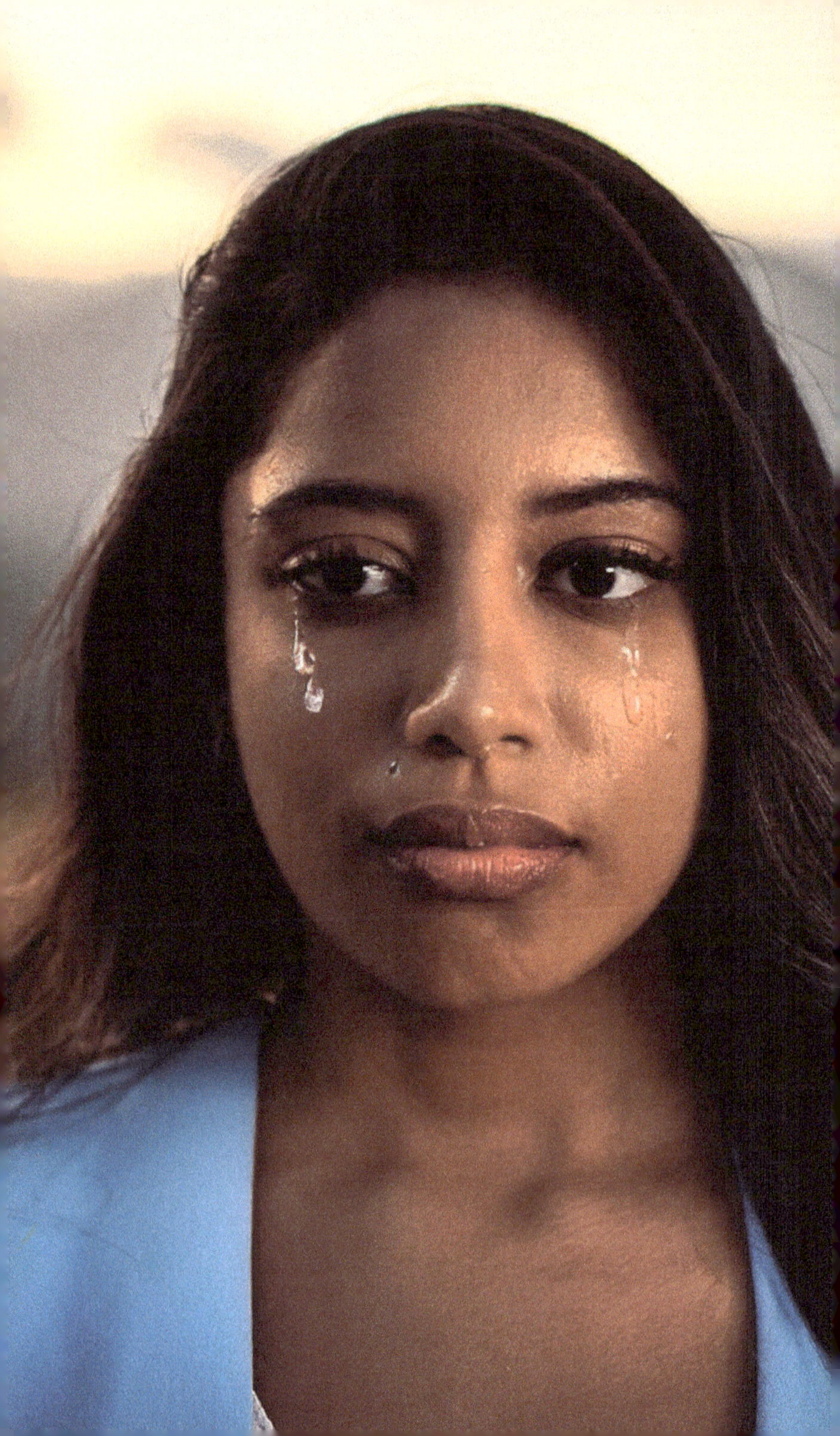

Crying

Welcome to Crying. Intentionally, crying is after Wading, and before Waiting. Why, you might ask? After years of examining empirical studies, and working with women and families, I have learned so much about brain development, especially our emotional wellness. The evolution of our fear responses - fight, flight, freeze, fawn – keeps our amygdala busy throughout our choices to survive, recover, and rebuild. It is our lived experiences that influence the way our autonomic nervous systems evidence our ability to adapt. In the big picture, over centuries, we have adapted to find food, shelter, kinship, and pleasure. Culturally, we have also adapted to thrive.

Having grown up in a family of strong women with many stories about our centuries of survival, I am fully aware of how biology has played its part in how I show my emotions. I am unapologetically aware of how physiological changes within my body can bring about physical responses to the meaning-making of stimuli. Simply put, my eyes tell stories about what my body is experiencing. Sometimes that shows up as joy, pain, anger, frustration, disbelief, resistance, and gratitude. Sometimes they share my light. I am convinced that wading in the water and experiencing the bonding of hydrogen and oxygen against my bronzed skin brings me balance.

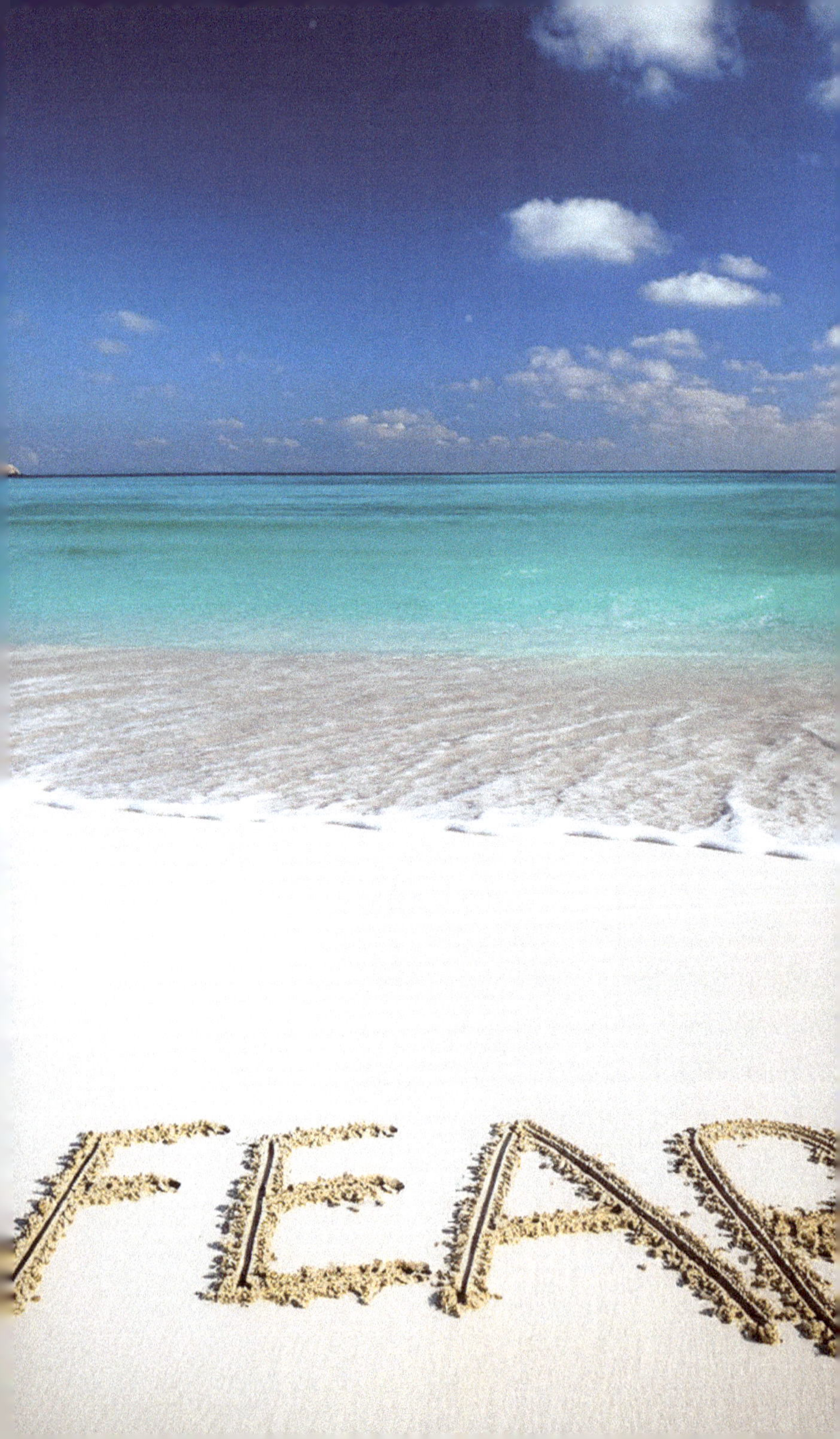

FEAR

I am convinced that my ancestors' tears and sweat are in the water that brings my feet relief and comfort.

I am not afraid to feel the comfort of my tears against my cheeks and I am comforted by the tears of my ancestors that flow in the water. I am comforted by the presence of their strength and courage that flows in the water. We are forever bonded by our blood, sweat, and tears.

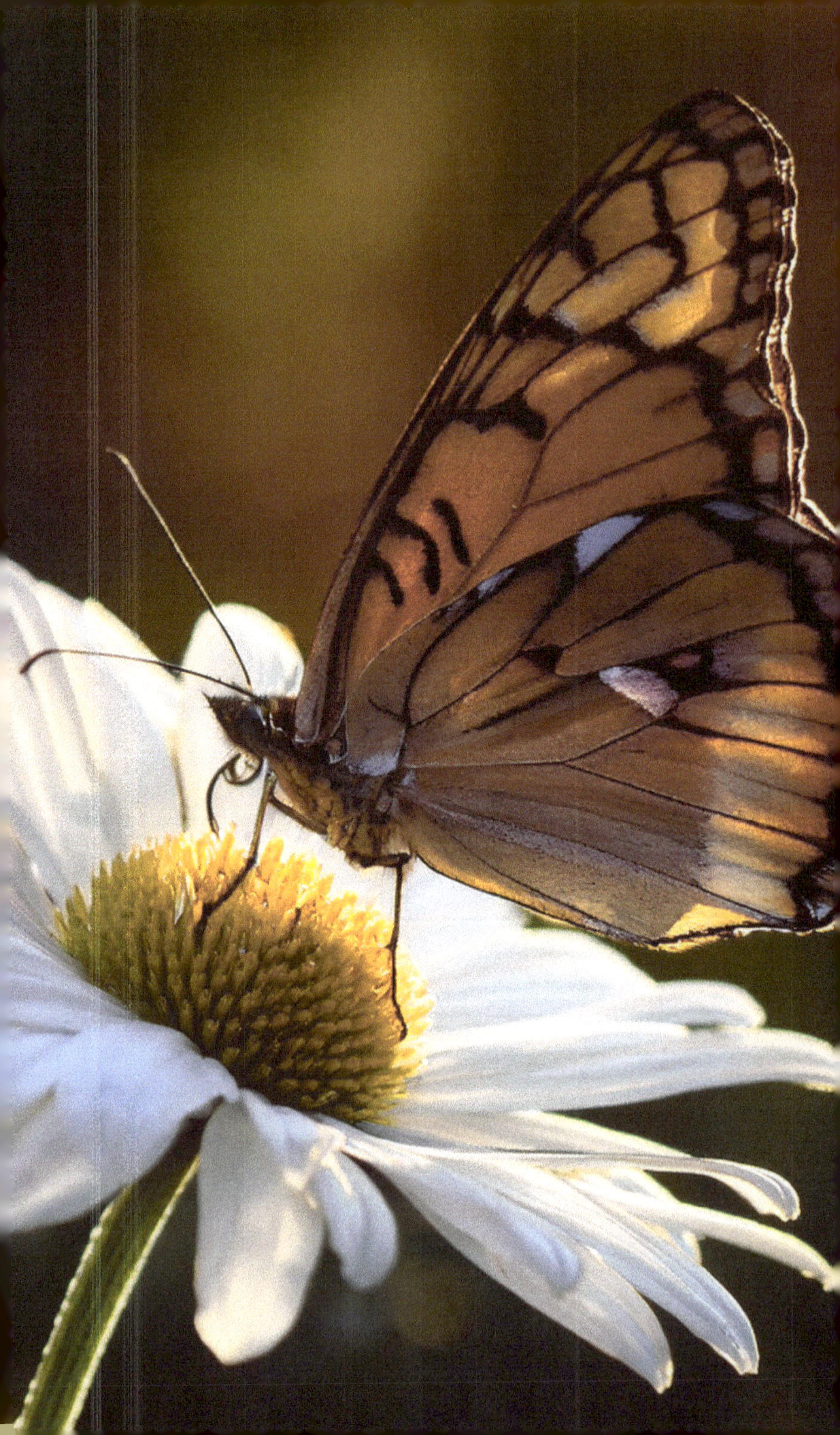

Waiting

Waiting can be difficult. Waiting requires us not only to pause and be still but to trust stillness and be brave enough to allow *Resilience* some rest. Sometimes waiting means we rely on others to help, support, and fill in for all things that matter. Sometimes waiting means we must trust others to pay the bills, prepare a meal, wash the clothes, care for our grandmother, water the plants, and even provide care for us. Sometimes waiting means praying for weeks and relying on a Higher Power, our God, to supply all of our needs. Sometimes waiting means we may actually take time to breathe, gaze, bathe, relax, and even visit Serenity. Sometimes it takes time to unlearn habits of constant doing and going. Our bodies may even resist the calm. Nevertheless, you are credible, capable, and creative, so do it anyway. Your sister *Resilience* will be grateful for an opportunity to visit her sister *Serenity*.

Intentionally be still.

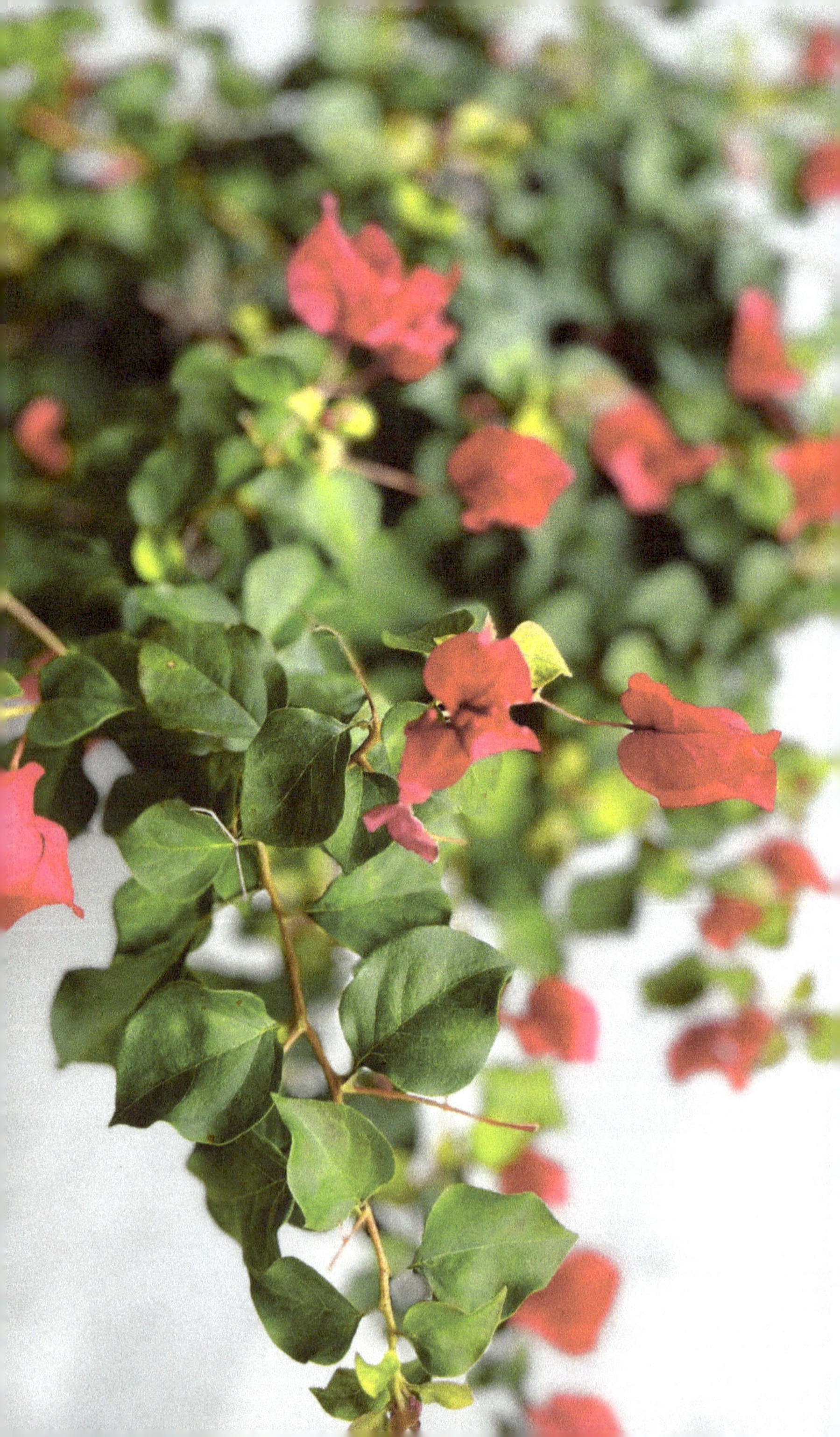

Intentionally pause to
smell the flowers.

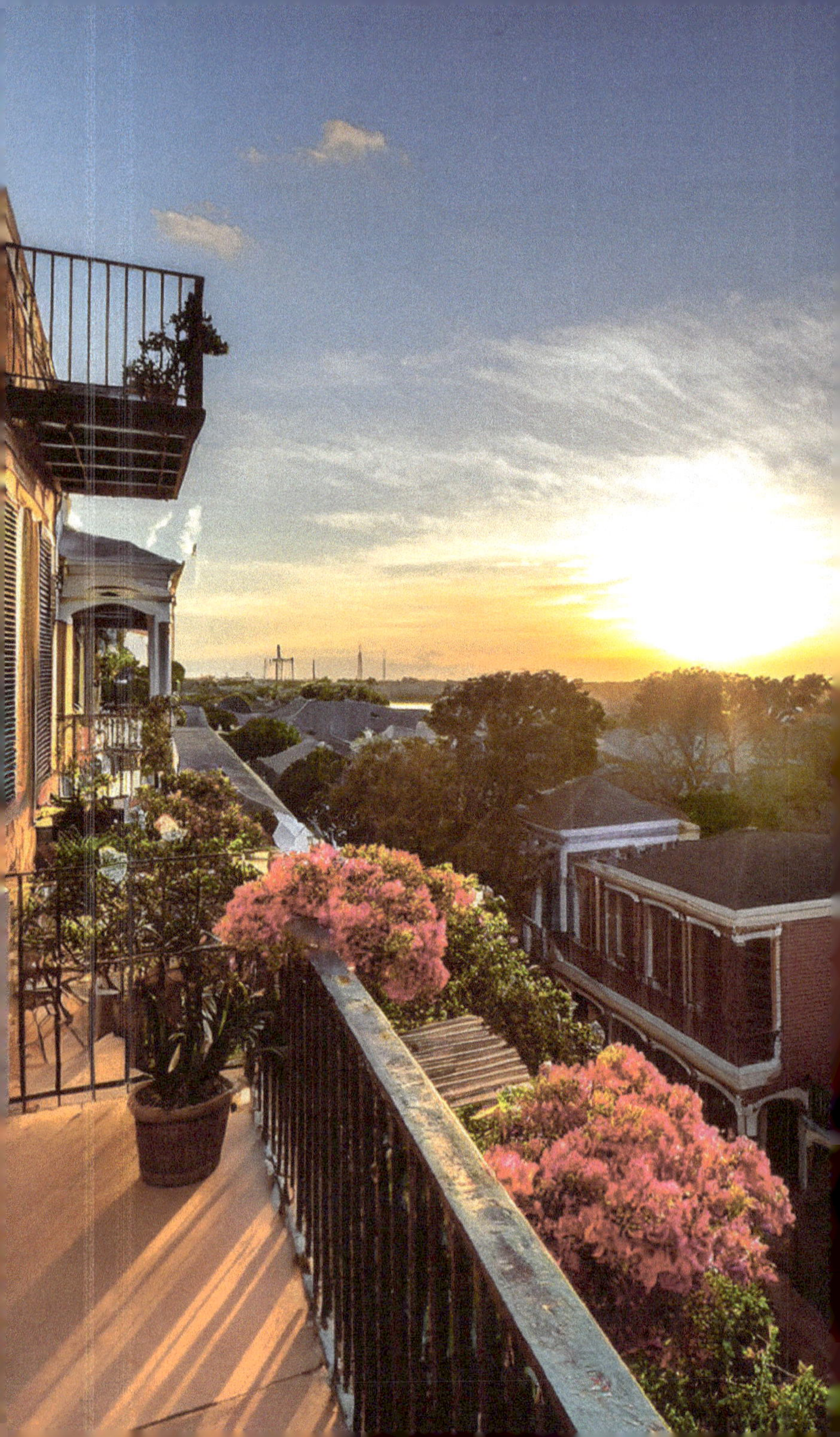

Lagniappe.

(a little something extra).

Intentionally gaze at a sunset.

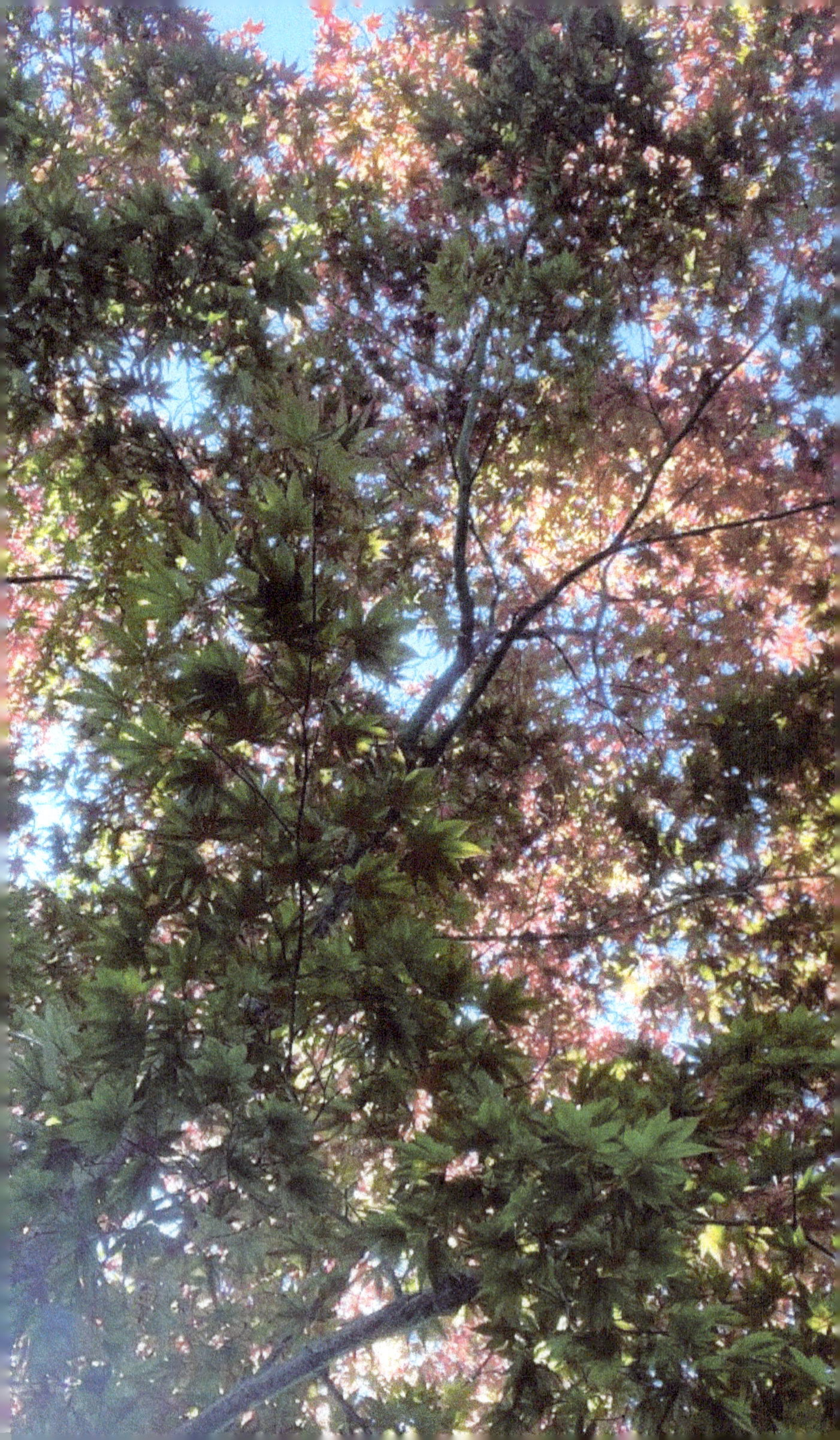

Look up.

Gaze at the trees.

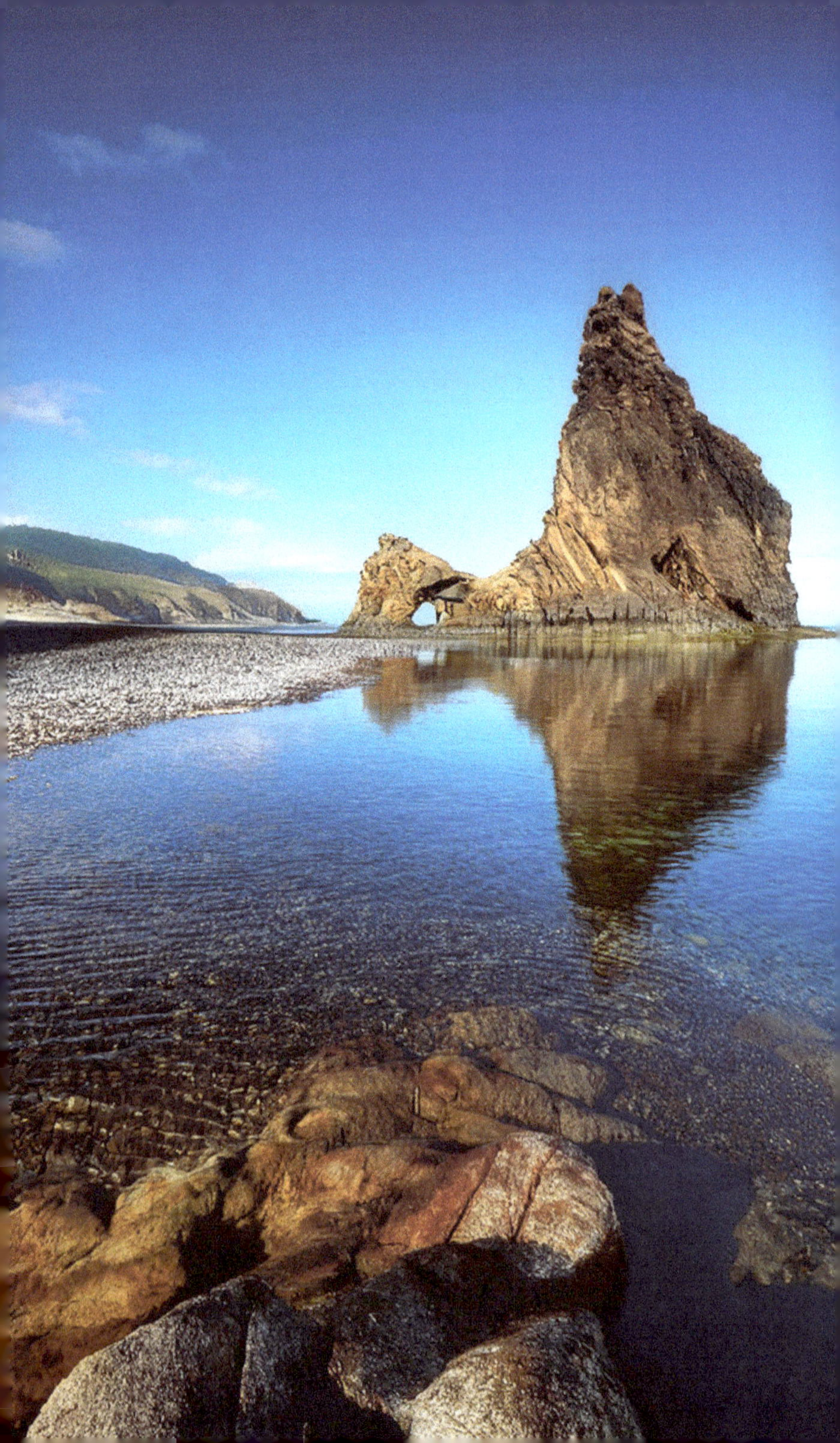

Conclusion

Wellness is a daily decision. Seeds of wellness must be cultivated regularly. Intentionally committing to practicing and sustaining healthy habits by maintaining a regimen that embraces Stillness is key. If you prioritize time for Stillness, your body will demonstrate longevity and reward you with wellness. I hope you choose to embody Stillness and enjoy a higher quality of life while thriving and giving your older sister, *Resilience*, a break.

About the Author

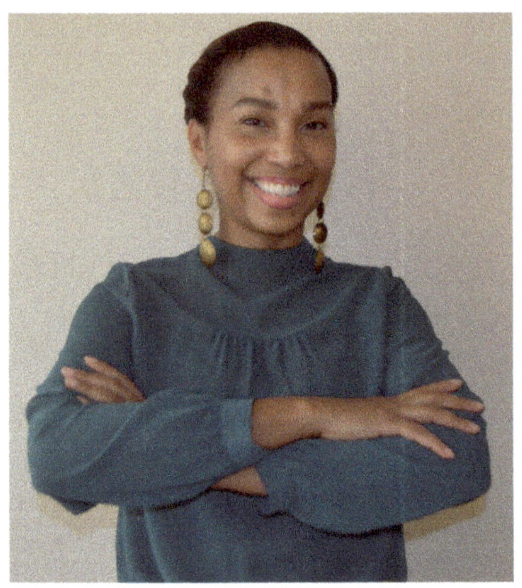

Maurya Walker Glaude

Maurya W. Glaude, Ph.D., M.S.W., L.C.S.W., BACS is a scholar-practitioner and artist who lives in the New Orleans area. She loves mentoring and teaching students as she prepares for the social work profession. Maurya is an active volunteer in her community, and she enjoys skating, painting, zydeco dancing, and traveling with family and friends.

For more support in your wellness journey, purchase the companion **Activity Guide - Stillness: 52 Weekly Activities to Rest, Relax, and Embody Wellness**.

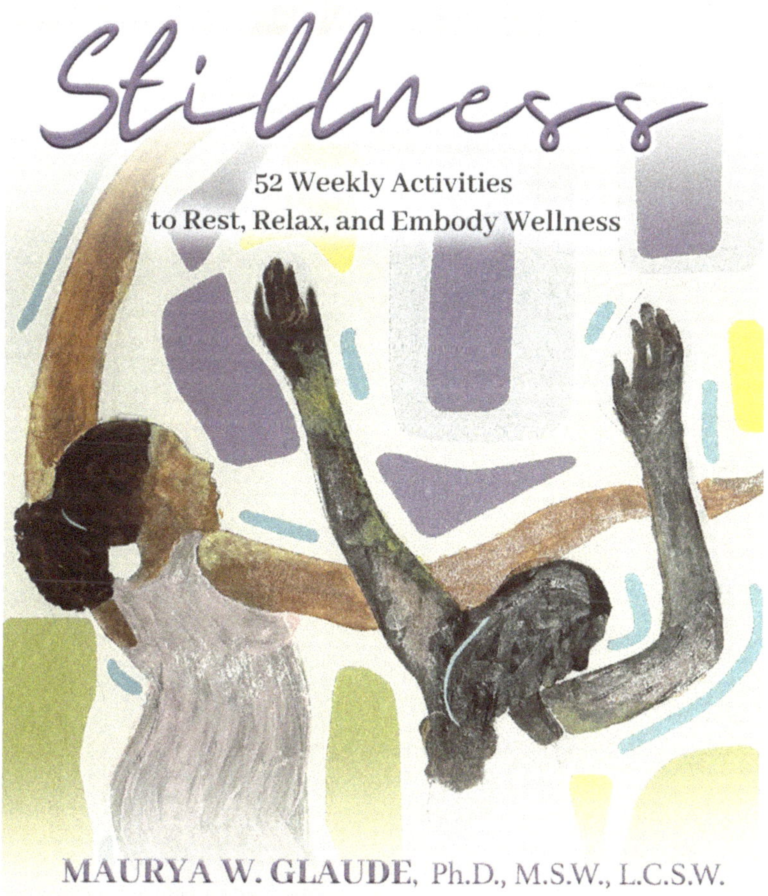

Paperback ISBN: 978-1-964972-02-2
Available everywhere books are sold.